LOCUST BEANS TO CURE CONJUNCTIVITIS

Exploring the Healing Powers of Locust Beans. A Natural Remedy for Conjunctivitis

Islamiyyah Fasasi

COPYRIGHT

TABLE OF CONTENTS

INTRODUCTION

Parkia biglobosa, the formal name for locust beans, is a type of leguminous plant indigenous to tropical Africa. They are also known as African locust beans, dawadawa, or iru in various African civilizations. They are members of the Fabaceae family. These beans are known for their unique scent, which is frequently described as nutty and pungent.

Trees that grow locust beans have elongated pods that carry seeds encased in a delicious pulp. The seeds are valuable in traditional medicine and culinary practices throughout Africa because of their high nutritional content and diverse medicinal characteristics.

CHAPTER ONE

Nutritional Composition of Locust Beans

Macronutrients

- Protein: With 20–30% protein by weight, locust beans are a major source of protein. They are a beneficial nutritional supplement because of their high protein content, particularly in areas with limited access to animal protein.

- Carbohydrates: Dietary fiber and sugars make up the majority of locust bean carbohydrates. While the sugars add to the pulp's sweet flavor around the seeds, the fiber content facilitates digestion and helps control blood sugar levels.

- Lipids: Although locust beans do not have a lot of fat, they do have some good fats, like monounsaturated and polyunsaturated fats, which are good for heart health.

Micronutrients

- Vitamins: B vitamins including thiamine (B1), riboflavin (B2), niacin (B3), and folate (B9), as well as vitamin C, are abundant in locust beans. These vitamins are vital for immunological response, energy metabolism, and general health.

- Minerals: Calcium, iron, magnesium, phosphorus, potassium, and zinc are among the many minerals found in locust beans. These minerals are essential for the body's numerous metabolic activities, blood flow, muscular contraction, and bone health.

Health Benefits

- Digestive Health: Regular bowel movements and the avoidance of constipation are made possible by the high fiber content of locust beans.

- Heart Health: By assisting in the regulation of blood pressure and cholesterol levels, heart-healthy fats, as well as vitamins and minerals like potassium, contribute to cardiovascular health.

- Immune Support: The vitamins and minerals present in locust beans are essential for bolstering the immune system and fending off illnesses and infections.

CHAPTER TWO

Medicinal Properties of Locust Beans

Antimicrobial Actions

The antimicrobial activity of locust beans is demonstrated against several bacteria, fungi, and other microbes. This characteristic is ascribed to substances present in locust beans, such as alkaloids, tannins, and flavonoids. Studies have demonstrated the potential of locust bean extracts to suppress the growth of harmful bacteria and fungi, so rendering them valuable for the management of illnesses.

Anti-inflammatory Properties

Locust beans are useful in lowering inflammation and its accompanying symptoms since they contain anti-inflammatory chemicals. Locust bean extracts are frequently used in traditional medicine to reduce inflammation-related pain, swelling, and redness, including dermatitis, arthritis, and gastrointestinal issues.

Antioxidants Contents

Antioxidants included in locust beans, such as vitamin C and phenolic compounds, help shield cells from oxidative damage brought on by free radicals. Antioxidants are essential for lowering the risk of long-term conditions like cancer, heart disease, and neurological illnesses. The general health-promoting effects of locust beans are partly attributed to their antioxidant capabilities.

Digestive Health

Traditionally, locust beans have been utilized to support and facilitate digestion and gastrointestinal health. Locust beans' high fiber content promotes healthy digestive function by preventing constipation and regulating bowel motions. Furthermore, locust bean chemicals may have gastroprotective qualities, which could aid in shielding the stomach lining and lessen the symptoms of gastrointestinal conditions like ulcers and gastritis.

Healing Wounds

Traditional medicine has used locust beans because of their possible ability to heal wounds. Locust bean extracts may hasten the healing of cuts, wounds, and abrasions while also encouraging the regeneration of skin tissue. Bioactive substances having anti-inflammatory and antibacterial qualities, which aid in tissue repair and infection prevention, are thought to be responsible for this impact.

Eye Health

Locust beans are used in various traditional medical practices to treat and prevent conditions connected to the eyes. Extracts from locust beans are thought to have calming and anti-inflammatory properties, which makes them useful for treating ailments like conjunctivitis, irritated eyes, and dry eyes. Ocular tissues are shielded from inflammation and inflammation by the presence of anti-inflammatory and antioxidant chemicals found in locust beans, which may be responsible for these effects.

Respiratory Health

Traditionally, locust beans have been utilized to improve respiratory health and ease symptoms related to the respiratory system. Locust bean extracts have the potential to alleviate coughs, lessen congestion, and lessen the signs and symptoms of respiratory diseases like asthma and bronchitis. The anti-inflammatory and antibacterial characteristics of locust beans, which aid in reducing respiratory tract inflammation and thwarting respiratory infections, are responsible for this respiratory-protective benefit.

CHAPTER THREE

Studies and Research on Locust Beans by Scientists

Clinical Trial Results and Analysis

Numerous clinical studies have been carried out to assess the potential health risks associated with locust bean consumption or its extracts. The effect of locust beans on variables like blood sugar, cholesterol, and inflammatory markers has been examined in this research. The results of these studies imply that including locust beans in the diet may improve cardiovascular risk factors, metabolic health, and general well-being.

Pharmacological Studies

The goal of the pharmacological study has been to clarify the modes of action and potential therapeutic applications of the bioactive substances present in locust beans. Numerous phytochemicals, including flavonoids, tannins, alkaloids, and phenolic compounds, have been found in locust beans through studies. These compounds have been shown to have pharmacological actions that include antibacterial, anti-inflammatory, and antioxidant properties. The potential application of these compounds in the creation of innovative therapeutic agents to treat a range of illnesses and ailments has been studied.

Nutritional Analysis

To learn more about the nutritional profile and possible health advantages of locust beans, nutritional studies have looked at their composition. According to this research, locust beans are an excellent source of important nutrients and antioxidants since they are high in protein, dietary fiber, vitamins, minerals, and bioactive compounds. When included in the diet, locust beans may help to promote health and fend off chronic diseases, according to nutritional assessments.

Bioavailability and Absorption

Studies have been carried out to evaluate the locust bean's bioavailability and absorption of nutrients and bioactive substances. Research has examined various aspects, including food matrix interactions, cooking methods, and processing and processing practices, that impact the nutrition that is absorbed, digested, and utilized from locust beans. Optimizing the nutritional impact and health advantages of locust beans requires an understanding of their bioavailability.

Safety and Toxicity Studies

To determine the safety and possible toxicity of locust beans and their extracts, safety evaluations have been carried out. Acute toxicity, genotoxicity, and allergenicity of locust beans have all been studied in order to verify that they are safe for ingestion by humans and use in medicine. Overall, studies show that locust beans are typically safe to eat in moderation, although further research is required to completely evaluate their safety profile.

CHAPTER FOUR

Application of Locust Beans in Modern Development

Formulation Development

Innovative formulators of food items, nutraceuticals, and medications are utilizing locust beans in their creations. They are adaptable ingredients that may be used to improve the nutritional value and sensory qualities of a variety of goods due to their distinct flavor character and nutritional makeup. To make use of locust beans' health advantages, products like protein-rich snacks, functional drinks, nutritional supplements, and medicinal preparations are being created.

Functional Foods and Beverages

Beans with locust characteristics are used to create functional foods and drinks that provide more than just basic nourishment. Goods like protein shakes, energy bars, herbal teas with locust bean extracts, and fortified cereals are becoming more and more popular with consumers who are concerned about their health. These functional meals and drinks are made to improve sports performance, promote general health, and deal with particular health issues like immune system support, digestive health, and cardiovascular well-being.

Applications in Pharmacies

Because of its possible therapeutic benefits and medical uses, locust beans are finding use in the pharmaceutical business. The antibacterial, anti-inflammatory, antioxidant, and other pharmacological properties of locust bean extracts are being studied. These bioactive substances have the potential to be used in the creation of novel medications and therapies for a range of illnesses and ailments, such as inflammatory diseases, infectious diseases, and chronic illnesses.

Cosmetic Formulations

Because locust beans have regenerating and skin-nourishing

qualities, they are employed in the development of cosmetics and personal care products. Locust bean extracts are used to protect, soothe, and hydrate the skin in skincare products like serums, lotions, and creams. Because locust beans are high in antioxidants, they can help prevent premature aging and oxidative stress, which makes them a useful component of natural skin care products and anti-aging formulas.

Agricultural Applications

Moreover, locust beans can be used in agriculture, especially for improving soil fertility and using sustainable farming methods. As nitrogen-fixing plants, locust bean trees enhance soil fertility and stimulate crop growth by adding nitrogen to the soil. Furthermore, locust beans can be applied as mulch, green manure, or organic fertilizers to improve soil structure, hold onto moisture, and inhibit weed growth. These applications support environmentally friendly farming practices and sustainable agriculture.

An alternative source of protein

Particularly in areas struggling with issues of food security and malnutrition, locust beans are becoming more and more recognized as a wholesome and sustainable alternative source of protein. Locust beans have a high protein content and an amino acid profile that makes them a viable plant-based protein source for human consumption. To meet the increasing demand for sustainable protein sources, products like protein bars, protein powders, and locust bean meat substitutes are being created.

Biodegradable Substances

Polysaccharides with sticky and gelling qualities, including galactomannans, are found in locust beans. Locust bean polysaccharides can be extracted and utilized to create biodegradable films, coatings, and packaging materials. These biodegradable materials support initiatives to lessen plastic pollution and environmental damage by providing a sustainable substitute for traditional plastics.

Production of Biofuel

As a sustainable and eco-friendly substitute for fossil fuels, locust beans can be used in the manufacturing of biofuels. Locust bean seeds have oil in them that can be collected and refined to create biodiesel, a sustainable fuel for diesel engines. The sustainability of locust bean farming can also be increased by using the byproducts of locust bean oil extraction, such as seed cake, as feedstock for anaerobic digestion, which produces biogas.

Value-Added Products

A variety of economically viable value-added products are being developed using locust beans. Gourmet foods like confections, handcrafted chocolates, and specialized condiments created with locust bean extracts are among these products. Furthermore, locust beans can be processed into components for industrial uses like stabilizers, thickeners, and adhesives, increasing their market potential and boosting the local economies of areas that produce locust beans.

Remediation of the Environment

There may be uses for locust beans in ecological restoration and environmental cleanup projects. Locust bean trees can flourish in arid or damaged environments because they are well-suited to a variety of environmental circumstances. They are ideal for reforestation, agroforestry, and land rehabilitation projects because of their deep root systems, which also serve to stabilize the soil, reduce erosion, and increase soil fertility. By utilizing locust beans' ecological advantages, these programs support biodiversity preservation and ecosystem restoration.

CHAPTER FIVE

Safety and Precautions

Allergic Reactions

Locust beans can cause allergic reactions in certain people, especially if they already have sensitivities to tree nuts or legumes. Locust bean allergies can cause rashes, itching, edema, respiratory problems, and gastrointestinal distress. People who are known to be allergic to locust beans should be cautious when eating them and should see a doctor if they have any negative responses.

Possible Adverse Reactions

Overindulging in locust beans or their extracts may cause adverse reactions like diarrhea, bloating, gas, or pain in the gastrointestinal tract. Locust beans should be consumed in moderation and one should be mindful of their own tolerance levels, particularly if they are being included in the diet for the first time.

Contraindications

When consuming locust beans, people who are pregnant, nursing, or on certain medications should proceed with caution. For instance, because locust beans are high in carbohydrates, individuals with diabetes should pay special attention to their blood sugar levels when consuming them. Furthermore, it is advisable to speak with a healthcare provider before consuming locust beans, particularly if you are taking prescription medicine, as they may interfere with certain medications.

Proper Preparations

Before consuming locust beans, they should be adequately cooked to guarantee their safety and flavor. Usually, this entails washing, dehusking, and occasionally heating or fermenting the beans to get rid of any anti-nutritional elements or possible contaminants. Additionally, in order to reduce the possibility of contamination or adulteration, locust beans must be sourced from reliable sources.

Storage and Handling

To keep them fresh and prevent spoiling, locust beans should be kept out of the heat, dampness, and sun. Instead, they should be kept in a cold, dry spot. The development of mold or bacteria that can cause foodborne diseases is impeded by proper storage. Additionally, in order to reduce the chance of contamination, locust beans should be prepared with hygiene in mind.

Pregnancy and Lactation

There is little information available on the safety of locust beans for women who are pregnant or nursing. Therefore, they should be consumed with caution. Although locust beans are usually regarded as safe to eat, women who are pregnant or nursing should speak with a healthcare provider to be sure they are a good fit for their particular situation before including them in their diet.

Hazardous Substances

Natural substances found in locust beans include alkaloids and tannins, which in excessive concentrations can be harmful. While these chemicals are normally found in low concentrations in locust beans and are not thought to be dangerous when ingested in moderation, excessive consumption may have negative consequences. Soaking, heating, or fermenting are examples of appropriate processing techniques that can lower the concentrations of harmful substances and improve the safety of locust beans for ingestion.

Children and Infants

When starting newborns and young children on locust beans, parents and other caretakers should proceed with caution. Although locust beans are healthy and advantageous for older kids, babies' developing digestive systems can make them more vulnerable to allergic responses or gastrointestinal distress. Before introducing locust beans to infants or young children, it is best to have a pediatrician check them to make sure they are developmentally mature and to address any concerns about possible allergies or intolerances.

Negative Outcomes:

Before ingesting locust beans, especially in large amounts or as part of concentrated extracts or supplements, those with underlying medical concerns such as kidney issues, autoimmune diseases, or gastrointestinal disorders should speak with a healthcare provider. It is imperative to see a doctor in order to prevent any issues as locust beans have the potential to worsen certain medical conditions or interfere with medications.

Purity and Quality

It is crucial to get locust beans or locust bean products from reliable suppliers who follow quality and safety guidelines. Make sure there are no additives, pesticides, or pollutants in the products. Verifying the quality and purity of locust bean goods and reducing the chance of exposure to hazardous materials can be achieved by carefully reading product labels and certificates.

Personal Hypersensitivity:

Although most people accept locust beans well, certain persons have different sensitivity levels or intolerances. After eating locust beans, some people may have gas, bloating, or pain in their digestive tracts, especially if they are not used to eating foods high in fiber. To prevent pain, it is critical to pay attention to your body and modify your locust bean consumption as necessary.

CHAPTER SIX

Cultivation and Harvesting of Locust beans

Regional Dispersion

The tropical portions of Africa, especially the Sahel region, which includes nations like Nigeria, Ghana, Senegal, and Mali, are home to locust bean trees. They grow well in savanna and semi-arid environments with lots of sunshine and well-drained soils.

Selection and Propagation of Seeds

Usually, the seeds of mature pods are used to grow locust bean trees. Farmers choose seeds from robust, healthy trees that exhibit desired qualities including consistent pod size, disease resistance, and high production. After that, the seeds are either spread directly in the field or in nurseries, where they sprout, develop into seedlings, and are subsequently moved to the final planting location.

Planting and Establishment

When soil moisture levels are sufficient for germination and establishment, locust bean trees are planted during the rainy season. The intended canopy size, water availability, and soil fertility are some of the variables that affect the distance between trees. Trees are usually planted 5–10 meters apart to provide sufficient ventilation and sunlight penetration.

Development and Sustaining

After they are established, locust bean trees do not need much care, although they do benefit from periodic trimming to get rid of unhealthy or dead branches and encourage strong development. To prevent weed development and preserve soil moisture, weed treatment, and mulching may also be required. To optimize land usage efficiency, farmers may occasionally employ intercropping techniques, growing different crops in between locust bean trees.

Fruit Development and Flowering

In general, locust bean trees start to bloom three to five years after planting, depending on the climate and overall health of the tree. The tiny, greenish-yellow blooms that the trees produce are clustered together and are pollinated by bees and butterflies. The blooms become lengthy pods after pollination, and it takes several months for them to ripen and mature.

Gathering

When locust bean pods are fully developed and ripe, they should be picked; color and texture changes are indicators of this. When the pods are ready to be harvested, they change from green to a yellowish-brown color and become slightly softer. using care to protect the trees and other pods, farmers painstakingly gather the pods using machetes or pruning shears. Harvested pods are gathered in sacks or baskets and taken to processing centers where they will receive additional care.

Handling

Locust bean pods are processed to separate the pulp and seeds after harvest. Usually, the pods are cracked open to extract the seeds, which are subsequently taken out of the pulp that surrounds them. Before being kept in storage or sold, the seeds can undergo additional processing such as roasting, fermenting, or drying. It is also possible to process the pulp that surrounds the seeds to create a variety of goods, including sauces, paste, and powdered locust beans.

Distribution and Storage

To keep their quality and shelf life, processed locust bean seeds and products are kept in cold, dry environments. After that, they are given to exporters, food processors, or local marketplaces for purchase and consumption. In many African nations, locust beans are a highly prized commodity that is employed widely in traditional medicine, gastronomy, and cultural rituals.

CHAPTER SEVEN

Sustainability and Preservation Activities.

Agroforestry and Reforestation

Through agroforestry programs and reforestation projects, efforts are being made to support the conservation and restoration of locust bean habitats. Restoring biodiversity, soil fertility, and ecosystem services can be achieved by planting locust bean trees in degraded or cleared regions. Locust bean trees in agroforestry systems with other crops offer a number of advantages, including shade, windbreaks, erosion control, and supplementary revenue streams for farmers.

Genetic Conservation

The goal of conservation initiatives is to maintain the genetic variety of locust bean trees by using ex-situ conservation techniques, seed banks, and germplasm collections. It is possible to preserve genetic resources and guarantee the availability of a variety of genetic materials for upcoming breeding and research projects by gathering and preserving seeds from several locust bean populations.

Sustainable Methods of Harvesting

In order to guarantee the locust bean trees' continuous output and regeneration, it is imperative to promote sustainable harvesting procedures. While satisfying consumer demand for locust beans, harvesting guidelines such as limiting the overexploitation of trees, allowing for natural regeneration, and selectively collecting mature pods help preserve healthy populations of locust bean trees.

Management in the Community

It promotes responsibility and a sense of ownership over natural resources when local communities are involved in the management and conservation of locust bean resources. Community-based projects provide local stakeholders the ability to apply sustainable land management techniques, take part in decision-making processes, and profit from the sustainable use of locust bean resources.

Awareness and Education

Promoting conservation efforts requires increasing public knowledge of the ecological significance of locust bean trees and the benefits of sustainable harvesting methods. Communities, decision-makers, and interested parties are educated about the advantages of preserving locust bean ecosystems and implementing sustainable land-use practices through educational programs, workshops, and outreach initiatives.

Support for Policy and Legal Protection

Enforcing rules and safeguarding locust bean ecosystems from hazards including deforestation, land degradation, and unsustainable land use practices require legislative backing and policy support. In order to give the preservation of locust bean trees and their ecosystems priority, governments and conservation organizations collaborate to create protected areas, conservation reserves, and land-use regulations.

Research and Monitoring

The main goals of research projects are to comprehend the biological dynamics of locust bean ecosystems, recognize the risks to their preservation, and create management plans that are sustainable. Monitoring programs keep tabs on shifts in biodiversity, habitat quality, and locust bean populations in order to evaluate the success of conservation efforts and direct adaptive management strategies.

CHAPTER EIGHT

Future Perspectives and Trends

Nutritional Security

Concerns about food security are driving up interest in plant-based protein sources as the world's population continues to rise. Because of their high protein content and nutritional value, locust beans have the potential to contribute significantly to addressing the growing need for wholesome, sustainable food sources, especially in areas where there is a problem with food insecurity.

Nutraceuticals and Functional Foods

The growing consumer desire for items that provide health advantages beyond basic nutrition is anticipated to fuel the growth of locust bean-based nutraceuticals and functional meals. Developments in formulation and food processing technology will open up new avenues for the production of dietary supplements, fortified foods, and functional food items with extracts from locust beans.

Sustainable Agriculture

Locust bean trees are prized for their contributions to agroforestry systems, enhancing soil fertility, and reducing the effects of climate change. Future agricultural trends are probably going to focus on sustainable farming methods, like conservation agriculture, agroforestry, and intercropping, which include locust bean trees into resilient and diverse farming systems.

Biorefinery and Value-Added Products

Technological developments in biorefineries will make it easier to use locust beans to produce high-value goods like biofuels, bioplastics, and biochemicals. The utilization of locust bean components, such as seeds, pulp, and husks, can optimize resource efficiency and enable the extraction of different products using biorefinery processes.

Pharmacological Investigations and Drug Finding

Further investigation into the therapeutic qualities of locust beans and their bioactive components could lead to the creation of novel medications and medical supplies. The goal of pharmacological research is probably to determine and describe the therapeutic potential of locust bean extracts to cure a range of illnesses and ailments.

Adaptation to Climate Change

Because locust bean trees thrive in semi-arid and drought-prone conditions, they are an important resource for efforts to adapt to climate change and increase resilience. Prospects for the future might include encouraging the use of locust bean trees in sustainable land management techniques and growing their cultivation in areas susceptible to climatic fluctuations.

Frameworks for Regulations and Policies

To encourage the sustainable use and protection of locust bean resources, regulatory and policy frameworks must be developed. Establishing rules, rewards, and regulations that promote ethical land management, biodiversity preservation, and fair access to locust bean resources will be a major task for governments, legislators, and international organizations.

CONCLUSION

To sum up, locust beans have long been known for their therapeutic qualities and medicinal qualities, which include the ability to lessen conjunctivitis symptoms. Because of its calming and anti-inflammatory qualities, locust beans have been used historically in traditional medicine to treat a variety of eye conditions, including conjunctivitis. Understanding the pharmacological characteristics of locust beans through scientific research has revealed their antibacterial, anti-inflammatory, and antioxidant capabilities. Because of these qualities, locust beans are a promising natural conjunctivitis treatment that can help alleviate irritation, lessen inflammation, and accelerate the healing of the damaged eye.

Locust beans also contain a wealth of nutrients, such as minerals, vitamins, and bioactive substances, all of which support general health and well-being. Beyond its potential to treat conjunctivitis, locust beans may also improve the digestive tract, immunological system, and cardiovascular health.

Although locust beans have shown promise as an adjunctive treatment for conjunctivitis, it is important to use caution when using them and seek medical advice from a professional to ensure appropriate diagnosis and treatment. People should also be aware of any allergies or sensitivities to locust beans, as well as any possible drug interactions.

In conclusion, locust beans have been used historically in traditional medicine, and new scientific evidence suggests that they may be a useful natural remedy for enhancing eye health and well-being. However, more research is required to completely understand the efficacy and mechanisms of action of locust beans in treating conjunctivitis.